Ketogenic Diet
A 14-Day Ketogenic Diet Plan For A Simple Start

Ken Davis

Copyright 2014 by Globalized Healing, LLC - All rights reserved.

Contents

WHAT IS KETOGENIC DIET? 1
WHY DO YOU NEED TO REDUCE CARBOHYDRATES IN THE DIET? ... 2
HOW PROTEINS AND FATS HELP? 3
BENEFITS OF KETOGENIC DIET 3
Success Plan for Ketogenic Diet 7
ABOUT THIS COOKBOOK 8
Day 1 11
Breakfast 11
    Spicy Scrambled Eggs 11
LUNCH 12
    Tuna Salad 12
DINNER 14
    Coconut Chicken Meatballs 14
    Grilled Peaches 16
DESSERT 17
    Healthy Dessert 17
Day 2 19
BREAKFAST 19
    Banana Pancakes 19
LUNCH 21
    Split Pea Soup 21
DINNER 23
    Kale and Pineapple Salad 23
SNACK 24
    Blueberry Juice 24

Ketogenic Diet: A 14-Day Ketogenic Diet Plan For A Simple Start

DESSERT	**26**
Pineapple bowl	26
Day 3	28
BREAKFAST	**28**
Honey Cinnamon Bread	28
LUNCH	**30**
Sweet & Sour Chicken	30
DINNER	**31**
Cheese Casserole	31
SNACK	**33**
Coconut Butter Stuffed Dates	33
DESSERT	**34**
Apple Crisp Dessert	34
Day 4	37
BREAKFAST	**37**
Breakfast Quinoa	37
Beef Roast with Potato	38
DINNER	**40**
Slow cooked Tomato Chicken	40
Banana and Tapioca Crepes	43
DESSERT	**44**
Blueberry Muffins	44
Day 5	47
Breakfast	47
Baked Salmon in the Breakfast	47
LUNCH	**49**
Mushroom, Tomato and spinach stir fry	49
DINNER	**51**
Dinner Steaks	51

SNACK	**53**
Honey Citrus Roasted Pecans	53
DESSERT	**55**
Blueberry Scones	55
Day 6	58
BREAKFAST	**58**
Strawberry Guava Smoothie	58
LUNCH	**59**
Baked Meatloaf	59
DINNER	**61**
Prawns Salad	61
SNACK	**63**
Fresh Fruit Bowl	63
DESSERT	**64**
Protein waffles	64
Day 7	67
BREAKFAST	**67**
Chicken Casserole	67
LUNCH	**68**
Salmon with Spinach & Apple Salad	68
DINNER	**70**
Roasted Beef with Vegetables	70
SNACK	**72**
Fruit Salad	72
DESSERT	**74**
Cherry and Almond Butter Milkshake	74
Day 8	76
BREAKFAST	**76**
Baked Omelette	76

Ketogenic Diet: A 14-Day Ketogenic Diet Plan For A Simple Start

Dinner **77**
    Mushrooms Soup 77
Snack **79**
    Kale Chips 79
Dessert **80**
    Pumpkin Muffins 80
Day 9 83
Breakfast **83**
    Omelette Chicken 83
Lunch **84**
    Roasted Fish with Bacon 84
Dinner **86**
    Grilled Chicken with Olives and Tomatoes 86
Snack **88**
    Green Smoothie 88
Dessert **89**
    Berries with Almonds 89
Day 10 91
Breakfast **91**
    Raspberry Almond Muffins 91
Lunch **93**
    Carrot Soup 93
Dinner **95**
    Fish Curry 95
Snack **97**
    Strawberry & banana Smoothie 97
Dessert **98**
    Apple Pudding 98
Day 11 100

BREAKFAST **100**
　Delicious Pancakes 100
LUNCH **101**
　Prawns with Tomato Sauce 101
DINNER **103**
　Sautéed Juicy Pork Tenderloin with Apple 103
SNACK **105**
　Banana Chips 105
DESSERT **106**
　Coconut Bread 106
Day 12 109
BREAKFAST **109**
　Jalapeno Scrambled Eggs with Cherry Tomatoes 109
LUNCH **111**
　Sautéed Leeks with Salmon 111
DINNER **112**
　Spicy Mixed Vegetable Curry 112
　Baked Apple 115
DESSERT **116**
　Coconut Whipped Cream 116
Day 13 118
Breakfast 118
　Eggs with Spicy Tomato Sauce ....
　.. 118
LUNCH **120**
　Thai Fish Curry 120
DINNER **122**
　Grilled Chicken with Olive and Tomato Topping 122
SNACK **124**

Watermelon & Kiwi with Fresh Herbs 124
DESSERT **125**
   Creamy Banana Treat with Cranberries and Coconut milk 125
Day 14 127
BREAKFAST **127**
   Breakfast Casserole 127
LUNCH **129**
   Grilled Spicy Beef 129
DINNER **130**
   Sweet & Salty Chocolate Bark 130
SNACK **132**
   Cocoa Almond Squares 132
DESSERT **133**
   Chocolate Pudding 133
Conclusion 135

Introduction

What is ketogenic diet?

The type of diet which is comparatively high in fat, adequate in protein and low in carbohydrates is known as ketogenic diet. This different combination changes the way of using the energy in the body. This diet is mainly used to achieve a metabolic state called ketosis. Ketosis is a state in which the human body burns and utilizes fat for the fuel needs instead of glucose and sugar. This normally happens when there is not enough glucose available. The fat is converted into ketones and fatty acids. The ketones are preferred by the brain to use as a fuel instead of the fatty acids. This is really very beneficial for the body. This helps the body to survive during the time interval when no or a little food is available. Nutritionists were also trying this ketosis state to cure many diseases like epilepsy, autism, Alzheimer's and different cancers.

Why do you need to reduce carbohydrates in the diet?

When you intake carbohydrates, you add to the glucose level in the blood forcing your pancreas to secrete insulin. The insulin is supposed to maintain the blood sugar to a certain level. To regulate the blood sugar the body uses insulin. It absorbs the extra glucose from the blood and stores it in the form of fats under the skin and around different organs as triglycerides. It also prevents those of the fat cells from breaking down and to be used as energy. It is interesting that this insulin acts as a guard for the body fats and to keep them from being used as energy. If you are taking sugar and sweets at a regular interval, then you are keeping your insulin level to a certain extent which keeps on storing glucose as fat. It also prevents your body fat to be released into the blood and to be used as energy which surely adds an extra pound of weight in a day or two. It is all about understanding the science of the body. If you want to release this extra fat of your body into the blood and use it as a source of energy, then you have to keep your insulin to as low as possible level. This is only possible if you reduce the amount of carbohydrates and sugars in your diet.

How proteins and fats help?

On the other hand, fats and proteins do not add a lot to the sugar level of the blood. The fats and proteins are made up of complex molecules and are not easy to be digested. Our body requires a large amount of energy to digest these fats and proteins. For this energy, the body depends on the fatty acids and ketone bodies. These fatty acids and ketones are produced by the liver using the fat stored in the body. In this way this diet can also work for the weight loss. The principle is the same, that is, to reduce the calorie intake and increase the need. This is how many nutritionists make different ketogenic diet plans for certain diseases like epilepsy.

Benefits of Ketogenic Diet

The ketogenic diet has many long term benefits like weight loss, cure from diseases and many others. In addition to these, this diet also offers a large number of everyday or common benefits which are listed below briefly.

- The best benefit of this ketogenic diet is that it provides freedom from hypoglycaemia and sugar cravings. It empowers you to not only have control over your diet and eating habits but also you enjoy being fit and healthy.
- This diet helps to decrease your hunger. It forces the body to depend on the fats stored in the body for the energy needs and the body learns how to survive when no food is available. You may realize at times that you forgot to eat but still feel no hunger.
- Ketogenic diet also helps to lower the blood pressure. This happens because all of the stored fat is converted into energy and is used by the body opening the veins and vessels of the blood wider, which might have been narrowed by the fat stored.
- Cholesterol is something which forms because of the excess glucose in the blood. It narrows the arteries and veins causing damage to the heart and brain. The brain gets the oxygen from the blood. High cholesterol makes the supply of the blood and oxygen to the brain difficult which

adds an extra pressure to the heart. This can cause heart attack and brain strokes which may result in the death. Cutting the carbohydrates in your diet reduces the glucose level in the blood. This helps to reduce the cholesterol and prevent many disorders and diseases.

- This diet helps you to feel more energetic. Instead of having a load of energy stored, you will actually have whole lot of energy. Protein is known for its muscle building properties. It also helps to repair damaged cells and tissues in the body. An adequate amount of energy will help you with muscle building at the same time when you are losing your extra fat. In short, this ketogenic diet is a complete package for a healthy life.

- This diet plan helps to reduce stiffness and joint pain. Just because it reduces the amount of fats stored in the body and provides a burst of energy, your muscles feel less stiffness. In addition the protein is there for the damage repair service and building new muscles.

- Our brain prefers to use the fatty acids as a source

of energy as compared to the glucose. Since this diet is based on fats and proteins which are a good source of fatty acids, so this diet is just like heaven for the brain. It helps you to have a clear thought and mind by making you feel fresh and energizing.

- This diet also helps to improve your digestion. You know that the fats and proteins are made up of the complex molecules and are not easy to digest. This digestion of proteins and carbohydrates helps the stomach and digestive system to strengthen.

Success Plan for Ketogenic Diet

There are many low carbohydrates and ketogenic diet plans from which you have to choose according to your needs and suitability. The basic idea, however, remains the same, that is, low carbohydrates, adequate protein and high fat.

This diet plan requires keeping an eye on the carbohydrates intake. You have to keep your carbohydrate intake between 40 to 60 grams per day. Any amount of carbohydrates between this range would be ideal. You may get the additional calories from the extra amount of fat you are going to add in the diet. You depend on fats for your 75 % of the calorie needs and 5 to 10 % on the carbohydrates.

To get started, first of all you have to know your needs and requirements and then you must have complete knowledge of the ketogenic diet. It is better to consult your nutritionists before adopting your diet. You need to go on a "carbohydrate sweep" in your house. Get rid of all the foods which are high in carbohydrates and replace them with those having high fat and proteins.

Replace your old habits with new and healthy ones. Whatever diet you are planning to adopt, keeping yourself hydrated is very necessary. More than 50% of the human body consists of water so it is very important part of any diet. The most important thing is to avoid the foods which you should not be eating and to keep yourself to derail for this healthy track. Firstly, you should plan, may be, 3 days of ketogenic diet to see whether it works for you or not. Or you may know the slight adjustments you need to make according to your ease. This book is a little effort to make you comfortable about this ketogenic diet. It consists of 14 days of meal plan of this amazing diet to set you on a new track of healthiness, fitness and happiness.

About This Cookbook

This cookbook is based on 14 days of ketogenic meal plan. The meal plan contains the amazing ketogenic breakfast recipes, lunch recipes, dinner recipes, snacks and dessert recipes for the whole day. These recipes are made for the common people and amateur chefs so that they can easily find a way to follow this diet plan. This cookbook will be a piece of cake for the professional chefs and people who know cooking. Along with the recipes, you will find serving size, preparation time, cooking time and the nutritional analysis for a confident start. The recipes are designed from the ingredients which are easily available in every market or superstore. The instructions are simple and easy to understand too. You simply need to have this cookbook and that is all for you to adopt this diet.

Day 1

Breakfast

Spicy Scrambled Eggs

Preparation time: 10 minutes   Cooking time: 5 minutes   Serves: 1

Ingredients

- 3 eggs
- 1 teaspoon cinnamon
- ¼ teaspoon ground allspice
- 1 tablespoon butter
- Pinch of salt

Directions

1. In a bowl, add eggs and beat until light.
2. Add in cinnamon and allspice and mix well.
3. Heat the butter in a non stick frying pan.
4. Add in eggs and cook for 1 minute.
5. Scramble the eggs using a wooden spatula.
6. Cook for 3-4 minutes more.

7. Sprinkle with salt and remove to a plate to serve.

Nutritional Information (for one serving)

Calories: 298

Fat Total: 24.7g

Fat Saturated: 11.4g

Carbohydrates: 3.2g

Dietary Fiber: 1.3g

Sugars: 1.1g

Protein: 16.9g

Lunch

Tuna Salad

Preparation Time: 5 minutes   Cooking Time: 0 minutes   Serves: 2

Ingredients:

- 1 avocado, mashed
- Juice of 1 lemon
- 1 can tuna, drained

- 1 tablespoon onion, chopped
- 1 tablespoon celery, chopped
- 1 tablespoon carrot, shredded
- Salt and pepper to taste
- 4 cups organic mix greens

Directions

1. In a bowl, combine mashed avocados with lemon juice.
2. Combine all the ingredients in it gently except the organic mix greens.
3. Season with salt and pepper.
4. Place mix greens onto a large plate, spoon tuna mixture on top and serve.

Nutritional Information (for one serving)

Calories: 715

Fat Total: 52.8g

Fat Saturated: 5.6g

Carbohydrates: 33.6g

Dietary Fiber: 11g

Sugars: 12.9g

Protein: 35.6g

Dinner

Coconut Chicken Meatballs

Preparation time: 20 minutes   Cooking time: 20 minutes   Serves: 6

Ingredients

- 1 cup zucchini, chopped
- 1 cup carrots, chopped
- ½ cup parsley, chopped
- 3 cloves garlic, minced
- ¼ cup coconut flour
- 1 egg, lightly beaten
- 1 pound boneless, skinless chicken breasts
- 1 teaspoon salt
- ½ teaspoon ground pepper
- ¼ teaspoon chili powder

Directions

1. Preheat the oven to 350 degrees F.

2. Place zucchini, carrots, parsley and garlic into a food processor and pulse.
3. Add in coconut flour, egg and chicken, salt and pepper and chili powder and pulse again until well combined.
4. Make 1 inch round shaped balls with your hands.
5. Place the meatballs onto greased parchment paper.
6. Bake in the oven for 20 minutes.
7. Remove from the oven and serve.

Nutritional Information (for one serving)

Calories: 190

Fat Total: 6.9g

Fat Saturated: 2g

Carbohydrates: 6.1g

Dietary Fiber: 2.6g

Sugars: 1.7g

Protein: 24.1g

Snack

Grilled Peaches

Preparation time: 15 minutes   Cooking time: 5 minutes   Serves: 4

Ingredients

- 4 medium peaches
- 2 tablespoons olive oil
- ¼ teaspoon ground cinnamon
- Pinch of ground cloves

Directions

1. Remove the pits from the peaches.
2. Add olive oil on the cut side of the peaches.
3. Sprinkle the peaches with cinnamon and cloves.
4. Place the peaches on the grill with medium heat and cut side down.
5. Grill for 5 minutes from the each side until softened.
6. Remove from the grill and let rest for 5 minutes before serving.

Nutritional Information (for one serving)

Calories: 99

Fat Total: 7.3g

Fat Saturated: 1g

Carbohydrates: 9.5g

Dietary Fiber: 1.6g

Sugars: 8.2g

Protein: 0.9g

Dessert

Healthy Dessert

Preparation time: 5 minutes   Cooking time: 0 minutes   Serves: 4

Ingredients

- 1 cup chopped walnuts, toasted
- 1 cup dried, unsweetened cherries

Directions

1. Combine together walnuts and cherries in a bowl and serve.

Nutritional Information (for one serving)

Calories: 214

Fat Total: 18.5g

Fat Saturated: 1.1g

Carbohydrates: 8.3g

Dietary Fiber: 2.2g

Sugars: 0 g

Protein: 7.6g

Day 2

Breakfast

Banana Pancakes

Preparation time: 15 minutes   Cooking time: 15 minutes   Serves: 2

Ingredients

- 1 egg
- 1 banana, mashed
- 1 teaspoon vanilla extract
- 2 tablespoons coconut flour
- Pinch of cinnamon
- ¼ teaspoon baking powder
- Pinch of sea salt
- Cooking spray

For Topping:

- ½ cup frozen mixed berries
- 1 tablespoon honey
- 2-3 tablespoons water

Directions

1. Place the egg in a bowl and beat until light.
2. Add mashed banana into the egg and mix.
3. Mix in vanilla extract.
4. Gradually add coconut flour, cinnamon, baking powder and salt into the bowl and mix until well combined.
5. Grease a non-stick frying pan lightly with the cooking spray.
6. Drop the mixture into the pan in portions.
7. Cook for 3-4 minutes for each side and remove to a plate.
8. Repeat the same instruction for the remaining mixture.
9. When the pancakes are cooking, place the mixed frozen berries in a saucepan with honey and water.
10. Heat the sauce pan until the berries are softened and come to a sauce like consistency.
11. Remove the pan from the heat and top the pancakes with this sauce for serving.

Nutritional Information (for one serving)

Calories: 145

Fat Total: 2.6g

Fat Saturated: 0.8g

Carbohydrates: 27.2g

Dietary Fiber: 3.1g

Sugars: 18.6g

Protein: 3.6g

Lunch

Split Pea Soup

Preparation time: 20 minutes   Cooking time: 3 hours   Serves: 6

Ingredients

- 1 tablespoon canola oil
- 1 onion, chopped
- 1 bay leaf
- 3 garlic cloves, minced
- 1 cup split peas, dried

- ¼ cup barley
- ½ tablespoon salt
- 4 cups water
- 2 carrots
- 1 celery stalks, chopped
- ½ cup parsley, chopped
- ½ teaspoon dried basil
- ½ teaspoon dried thyme
- ½ teaspoon ground black pepper

Directions

1. In a large pot, add the canola oil and heat.
2. Add in onion, bay leaf and garlic and cook for 4-5 minutes.
3. Add peas, barley, salt and water.
4. Cover and cook for 2 hours until peas are well cooked and soft.
5. Remove the lid and add carrots, celery, potatoes, parsley, basil, thyme and black pepper.
6. Cover and cook for one hour more.
7. When all the vegetables are well cooked, remove

from the heat and serve.

Nutritional Information (for one serving)

Calories: 181

Fat Total: 3g

Fat Saturated: 0g

Carbohydrates: 30g

Dietary Fiber: 10.9g

Sugars: 4.6g

Protein: 9.6g

Dinner

Kale and Pineapple Salad

Preparation Time: 15 minutes   Cooking Time: 25 minutes   Serves: 3

Ingredients

- 1 medium kale, de-stemmed and shredded
- 2 tablespoons olive oil
- 3 parsnips, shredded
- 1 cup pineapple, cut into cubes

- Sea salt and black pepper, to taste

Directions

1. In a large bowl, add kale and olive oil.
2. Add in parsnips and pineapple and toss well.
3. Sprinkle with salt and black pepper and serve.

Nutritional Information (for one serving)

Calories: 107

Fat Total: 9.4g

Fat Saturated: 1.3g

Carbohydrates: 7.2g

Dietary Fiber: 0.8g

Sugars: 5.4g

Protein: 3g

Snack

Blueberry Juice

Preparation time: 5 minutes   Cooking time: 0 minutes   Serves: 3

Ingredients

- 2 cups blueberries
- 1 cup fresh strawberries
- 1 tablespoon lemon juice
- 2 small apples, peeled and diced
- 1½ cup baby spinach
- 1 carrot, sliced

Directions

1. Add all the ingredients into a juicer and pulse.
2. Pour the juice into glasses and serve chilled.

Nutritional Information (for one serving)

Calories: 135

Fat Total: 0.7g

Fat Saturated: 0g

Carbohydrates: 34.1g

Dietary Fiber: 6.6g

Sugars: 23.4g

Protein: 1.9g

Dessert

Pineapple bowl

Preparation time: 10 minutes   Cooking time: 0 minutes   Serves: 3

Ingredients

- ½ of a ripe pineapple, peeled and cored
- Salt and cayenne pepper, to taste
- 2 tablespoons fresh mint leaves, chopped
- 2 tablespoons fresh coriander leaves, chopped

Directions

1. Make bite-sized slices of pineapple. In a bowl, add pineapple, mint and coriander leaves and combine.
2. Season with salt and cayenne pepper and serve.

Nutritional Information (for one serving)

Calories: 29

Fat Total: 0.1g

Fat Saturated: 0g

Carbohydrates: 7.6g

Dietary Fiber: 1.1g

Sugars: 5.4g

Protein: 0.4g

Day 3

Breakfast

Honey Cinnamon Bread

Preparation time: 20 minutes   Cooking time: 30 minutes   Serves: 4

Ingredients

- 3 eggs
- 2 tablespoons honey
- 1 teaspoon vanilla extract
- 2 tablespoons coconut oil
- 1 cup almond flour
- 1 tablespoon cinnamon
- Pinch of sea salt
- ¼ cup raisins
- 2 tablespoons walnuts, chopped

Directions

1. Preheat the oven to 350 degrees F.
2. In a bowl, add eggs and beat until light.

3. Add in honey, vanilla extract and coconut oil and mix again.
4. Whisk together almond flour, cinnamon and salt in another bowl.
5. Gradually, add the flour mixture into the bowl with the liquid mixture and mix until smooth dough is formed.
6. Mix in raisins.
7. Pour the mixture into a greased 8x8 inch bread pan and spread chopped walnuts over the surface of the dough.
8. Bake in the oven for 25-30 minutes.
9. Remove from the oven and set aside to cool.
10. Cut into slices and serve.

Nutritional Information (for one serving)

Calories: 196

Fat Total: 12.4g

Fat Saturated: 7g

Carbohydrates: 18g

Dietary Fiber: 1.5g

Sugars: 14.4g

Protein: 5.5g

Lunch

Sweet & Sour Chicken

Preparation time: 15 minutes   cooking time: 30 minutes   serves: 4-5

Ingredients

- 1 pound skinless and boneless chicken, cut into chunks
- 3 tablespoons olive oil
- 1 fresh orange, peeled and squeezed
- Zest of 1 orange
- 1 tablespoon lemon juice
- 1 teaspoon fresh grated ginger
- 3 tablespoons coconut amino
- ½ cup chopped scallions

Directions

1. Heat the olive oil in a sauce pan.
2. Add chicken and cook until browned.

3. Meanwhile, add orange juice, orange zest, lemon juice, ginger and coconut amino in a saucepan and cook.
4. Add the browned chicken into the sauce when it gets thickened.
5. Stir and cook for 5-7 minutes.
6. Remove from the heat and serve.

Nutritional Information (for one serving)

Calories: 255

Fat Total: 12g

Fat Saturated: 1.6g

Carbohydrates: 7.5g

Dietary Fiber: 1.5g

Sugars: 4.7g

Protein: 35.4g

Dinner

Cheese Casserole

Preparation time: 25 minutes   cooking time: 50

minutes   serves: 4-5

Ingredients

- 1 medium eggplant, sliced
- 8 ounce mozzarella cheese, shredded
- 5 ounce parmesan, shredded
- 1 pound sausage scramble, cooked
- 8 ounce marinara
- 1 tablespoon olive oil

Directions

1. Preheat the oven to 375 degrees F.
2. Grease a baking dish with the olive oil.
3. Place the eggplant slices in the baking dish.
4. Spread half of the marinara over the eggplants.
5. Spread half of the mozzarella and parmesan over and top with sausages scramble.
6. Spread the remaining half of mozzarella and parmesan.
7. Top with marinara and sprinkle some salt and pepper.
8. Bake in the oven for 50 minutes.

Nutritional Information (for one serving)

Calories: 417

Fat Total: 28.4g

Fat Saturated: 13.6g

Carbohydrates: 11.4g

Dietary Fiber: 3.7g

Sugars: 3.6g

Protein: 30.2g

Snack

Coconut Butter Stuffed Dates

Preparation time: 10 minutes   cooking time: 0 minutes   serves: 4

Ingredients

- 8 dates
- ¾ cup coconut butter
- ¼ teaspoon of cinnamon

Directions

1. Remove the pits from the dates and place in a

bowl.
2. Mix the cinnamon with the coconut butter.
3. Using a spoon, add the butter into the dates one by one and serve.

Nutritional Information (for one serving)

Calories: 103

Fat Total: 5.4g

Fat Saturated: 4.8g

Carbohydrates: 14.6g

Dietary Fiber: 2.9g

Sugars: 11g

Protein: 0.9g

Dessert

Apple Crisp Dessert

Prep-time: 1 hour 10 minutes   Cooking time: 35 minutes   Serves: 8

Ingredients

- 4 medium apples, peeled, cored and sliced thinly

- 1 tablespoon lemon juice
- 1½ cup almond flour
- 1 tablespoon cinnamon
- 4 tablespoons honey
- 4 tablespoons almond oil
- 2 tablespoons sugar
- Pinch of salt

Directions:

1. Preheat the oven to 325 degrees F.
2. Grease an 8x8 inch baking dish.
3. Place the apple slices in the dish and spread evenly.
4. Drizzle lemon juice over the apple slices and set aside.
5. In another bowl, add almond flour, cinnamon, honey, almond oil and sugar and mix until well combined.
6. Spread the mixture over apples and spread evenly.
7. Place the dish in the oven and bake for 30-35

minutes.

8. Remove from the oven and serve.

Nutritional Information (for one serving)

Calories: 183

Fat Total: 9.6g

Fat Saturated: 0.8g

Carbohydrates: 26.1g

Dietary Fiber: 3.2g

Sugars: 21.3g

Protein: 1.4g

Day 4

Breakfast

Breakfast Quinoa

Preparation time: 15 minutes   Cooking time: 30 minutes   Serves: 4-6

Ingredients

- 2 cups low-fat milk
- 3 tablespoons honey
- 1 cup quinoa, rinsed
- 1/8 teaspoon cinnamon, ground
- 1 cup fresh blueberries

Directions

1. In a saucepan boil milk, add quinoa and again bring it to a boil.
2. Reduce heat and let it simmer covered for about 15 minutes.
3. Now stir in honey and cinnamon and cook covered again for about 8 minutes or until all the milk is almost absorbed.

4. Drop in blueberries and cook for just 30 seconds.
5. You can serve it with additional milk and blueberries.

Nutritional Information (for one serving)

Calories: 214

Fat Total: 3g

Fat Saturated: 0.8g

Carbohydrates: 40g

Dietary Fiber: 3g

Sugars: 18.3g

Protein: 8.1g

Lunch

Beef Roast with Potato

Preparation time: 15 minutes   Cooking time: 2 hours 40 minutes   Serves: 10

Ingredients

- 2 large potatoes, peeled and sliced

- 1 large onion, cut into thick wedges
- 3 pounds grass-fed bottom round beef roast
- 8 garlic cloves, minced
- Sea salt and black pepper, to taste
- 12 fresh sage leaves, chopped
- 1 cup of beef broth

Directions

1. Preheat the oven to 350 degrees F.
2. In a large baking dish, place the beef in the middle of the dish.
3. Place the potatoes and onion around the roast.
4. Using a sharp knife, make slices in the roast all around.
5. Place the minced garlic in the slices. Pour the beef broth over the roast.
6. Cover with the foil and roast in the oven for 2 hours.
7. Remove the foil and roast again for 30-40 minutes.
8. Remove from the heat and serve.

Nutritional Information (for one serving)

Calories: 357

Fat Total: 11.7g

Fat Saturated: 4g

Carbohydrates: 15.3g

Dietary Fiber: 3.1g

Sugars: 1.6g

Protein: 45.2g

Dinner

Slow cooked Tomato Chicken

Preparation time: 20 minutes   Cooking time: 5 hours 20 minutes   Serves: 6

Ingredients

- 1 pound boneless and skinless chicken breasts
- ½ teaspoon sea salt
- ¼ teaspoon ground black pepper
- 1 tablespoon coconut oil
- ½ cup diced red pepper

- ½ cup diced zucchini
- 1 cup sliced carrots
- 1½ cup cubed sweet potatoes
- ½ yellow onion, diced
- 1 (15 ounce) can diced tomatoes
- 1 (15 ounce) can crushed tomatoes
- 8 tablespoons tomato paste
- 3 tablespoons balsamic vinegar
- 3 garlic cloves, minced
- 1 tablespoon dried oregano
- ¼ teaspoon red pepper flakes
- 2 sprigs of fresh rosemary
- 2 sprigs fresh thyme
- ¼ cup chopped fresh basil

Directions

1. Heat the coconut oil in a non-stick skillet.
2. Sprinkle chicken breasts with salt and pepper and add into the pan.
3. Cook from both sides until browned.

4. Remove from the heat and shred when cooled completely.
5. Add chicken, red pepper, zucchini, carrots, sweet potatoes, onion, diced and crushed tomatoes, balsamic vinegar, cloves, oregano, red pepper flakes, rosemary, thyme and basil in a slow cooker and mix until combined.
6. Cover and cook for 4-5 hours.
7. Remove from heat and stir before serving.

Nutritional Information (for one serving)

Calories: 225

Fat Total: 3.7g

Fat Saturated: 2g

Carbohydrates: 27.5g

Dietary Fiber: 6.9g

Sugars: 10.5g

Protein: 22g

Snack

Banana and Tapioca Crepes

Preparation time: 20 minutes   Cooking time: 25 minutes   Serves: 8

Ingredients

- 5 ripe bananas, peeled
- 6 organic eggs
- 1½ cup organic coconut milk
- ½ teaspoon ground cinnamon
- 1 teaspoon sea salt
- 2 cups tapioca flour

Directions

1. Place the bananas in a bowl and mash with a fork.
2. In another bowl, add eggs, one by one, and beat until light and fluffy.
3. Add in mashed bananas, sea salt, cinnamon and mix.
4. Gradually add flour and mix until smooth dough is formed.
5. Heat a non-stick pan.

6. Pour ¾ -1 cup of batter into the pan.
7. Cook for 3-4 minutes or until golden brown.
8. Flip and cook from the other side for 3-4 minutes.
9. Remove from the pan and repeat the process.

Nutritional Information (for one serving)

Calories: 312

Fat Total: 14g

Fat Saturated: 10.6g

Carbohydrates: 42.2g

Dietary Fiber: 3.5g

Sugars: 10.5g

Protein: 5.9g

Dessert

Blueberry Muffins

Preparation time: 25 minutes   Cooking time: 20 minutes   Serves: 8

Ingredients

- 2 organic eggs
- 1 cup butter
- ½ cup raw honey
- ¼ cup olive oil
- ¼ cup shredded coconut, unsweetened
- 1 cup coconut flour
- 1 teaspoon baking powder
- ¼ teaspoon sea salt
- ¼ teaspoon cinnamon
- ½ cup fresh blueberries

Directions

1. Preheat the oven to 350 degrees F.
2. In a large bowl, add eggs and beat until light.
3. Add in butter and beat again.
4. Mix in honey and olive oil and set aside.
5. In another bowl, combine coconut, coconut flour, baking powder, sea salt and cinnamon.
6. Gradually add into eggs and butter mixture and mix.

7. Add in blueberries and mix until well combined.
8. Pour the mixture into the greased muffins pan.
9. Bake in the oven for 15-20 minutes.
10. Remove from the heat and let cool completely before serving.

Nutritional Information (for one serving)

Calories: 414

Fat Total: 17.1g

Fat Saturated: 17.1g

Carbohydrates: 27.6g

Dietary Fiber: 5.5g

Sugars: 19.5g

Protein: 3.8g

Day 5

Breakfast

Baked Salmon in the Breakfast

Preparation time: 10 minutes   Cooking time: 40 minutes   Serves: 2

Ingredients

- 2 tablespoons coconut oil
- 2 (4 ounces each) salmon fillets
- 2 teaspoons dried thyme
- 1 teaspoon garlic powder
- 3 teaspoons dried dill
- ¼ teaspoon salt
- ¼ teaspoon paprika powder

Directions

1. Preheat the oven to 350 degrees F.
2. Add 1 tablespoon of coconut oil into a baking dish to grease.
3. Place the salmon into the baking dish and driz-

zle the remaining coconut oil over them.

4. In a small bowl, add thyme, garlic powder, dried dill, salt and paprika and mix.
5. Sprinkle the thyme and garlic mixture over the fillets.
6. Bake in the oven for 18-20 minutes.
7. Remove from the oven and serve.

Nutritional Information (for one serving)

Calories: 278

Fat Total: 20.8g

Fat Saturated: 12.8g

Carbohydrates: 2.5g

Dietary Fiber: 0.7g

Sugars: 0g

Protein: 22.6g

Lunch

Mushroom, Tomato and spinach stir fry

Preparation time: 20 minutes   Cooking time: 30 minutes   Serves: 4

Ingredients

- 1 teaspoon vegetable oil
- 6 button mushrooms, sliced
- 2 tablespoons olive oil
- Half red onion, sliced
- ¼ cup cherry tomatoes, halved
- 1 teaspoon lemon zest
- 1 clove garlic, minced
- ½ teaspoon sea salt
- Pinch of black pepper, grounded
- Pinch of nutmeg
- 3 handfuls of spinach
- 1 tablespoon lemon juice

Directions

1. Add the vegetable oil in a large pan and heat.

2. Add in mushrooms and sauté for 4 minutes.
3. Remove to a plate when the mushrooms are browned.
4. Add the olive oil into the same pan and heat.
5. Add onion and cook for 3-4 minutes.
6. Add in tomatoes, lemon zest and garlic.
7. Stir and cook and stir for 4 minutes.
8. Sprinkle sea salt, pepper and nutmeg.
9. Add in spinach and cook until spinach is wilted.
10. Remove to a plate and drizzle with lemon juice.

Nutritional Information (for one serving)

Calories: 358

Fat Total: 16.5g

Fat Saturated: 5.8g

Carbohydrates: 42.2g

Dietary Fiber: 8g

Sugars: 3.8g

Protein: 13g

Dinner

Dinner Steaks

Preparation time: 25 minutes   Cooking time: 55 minutes   Serves: 4

Ingredients

- 1 pound grass-fed beef
- 2 shallots, minced
- 1 egg yolk, beaten
- ½ teaspoon sea salt
- ½ teaspoon ground black pepper
- 2 tablespoons olive oil
- For Sauce:
- 1 cup beef stock
- ½ cup apple cider vinegar
- 3 sprigs fresh thyme, chopped
- ¼ cup butter
- ¾ pound porcini mushrooms, washed and coarsely chopped
- 1 yellow onion, sliced

Directions

1. In a large bowl, add shallots, egg yolk, sea salt and black pepper and olive oil and mix.
2. Slice the beef into four equally sized steaks and toss with shallots mixture. Set aside.
3. Pour beef stock and vinegar in a large skillet and bring to a boil.
4. Add in thyme and cook until it is reduced to half.
5. Heat 2 tablespoons of butter in a saucepan. Add mushrooms and sauté for 3-4 minutes.
6. Remove from the pan and add in yellow onion.
7. Sauté onion for 5 minutes or until translucent.
8. Remove from the heat.
9. In a non-stick saucepan, heat 2 tablespoons of butter until melted.
10. Add the steaks one by one and cook for 3-4 minutes from each side.
11. Cook the remaining steaks following the same procedure.

12. Remove in serving plates with yellow onion and mushrooms.
13. Drizzle prepared sauce over and serve.

Nutritional Information (for one serving)

Calories: 679

Fat Total: 25.9g

Fat Saturated: 10.8g

Carbohydrates: 45.7g

Dietary Fiber: 21.9g

Sugars: 1.3g

Protein: 48.3g

Snack

Honey Citrus Roasted Pecans

Preparation time: 10 minutes   Cooking time: 30 minutes   Serves: 4-6

Ingredients

- 6 ounce raw pecans
- 3 tablespoons raw honey

- Pinch of sea salt
- 1 teaspoon orange zest, minced
- Pinch of ginger powder

Directions

1. Preheat the oven to 350 degrees F.
2. Place the pecans in a baking sheet lined with parchment paper in the form of a single layer.
3. Bake for 10-12 minutes.
4. Meanwhile, combine honey, sea salt, orange zest and ginger powder in a bowl.
5. Remove the nuts from the oven and add into the honey mixture.
6. Toss until nuts are well combined.
7. Place the nuts again on the baking sheet.
8. Bake for 15-20 minutes.
9. Remove from the oven and serve when cooled completely.

Nutritional Information (for one serving)

Calories: 276

Fat Total: 24.3g

Fat Saturated: 2.4g

Carbohydrates: 15.4g

Dietary Fiber: 3.7g

Sugars: 11.6g

Protein: 3.7g

Dessert

Blueberry Scones

Preparation time: 40 minutes   Cooking time: 15 minutes   Serves: 6

Ingredients

- 1 egg
- ¼ cup honey
- 1 tablespoon vanilla extract
- 2½ cups coconut flour
- 2 tablespoons arrowroot powder
- 1 teaspoon baking powder
- ½ teaspoon salt
- ½ cup frozen blueberries

Directions

1. Preheat the oven to 350 degrees F.
2. In a large bowl, add egg and beat until light.
3. Add in honey and vanilla extract and beat again.
4. Add coconut flour, arrowroot powder, baking powder and salt and mix until smooth dough is formed.
5. Add in blueberries and mix again.
6. Shape the dough into a ball and place onto a baking sheet lined with parchment paper.
7. Flatten the ball to about ½ inch thickness and cut into slices like a pizza.
8. Bake in the oven for 12-15 minutes.
9. Remove from the heat and serve when cooled.

Nutritional Information (for one serving)

Calories: 286

Fat Total: 5.8g

Fat Saturated: 1.9g

Carbohydrates: 43.4g

Dietary Fiber: 17g

Sugars: 16.4g

Protein: 7.7g

Day 6

Breakfast

Strawberry Guava Smoothie

Preparation time: 15 minutes   Cooking time: 0 minutes   Serves: 2

Ingredients

- 1 cup strawberries, quartered
- 1 (6 ounce) can of strawberry fat-free yogurt
- 1 banana, sliced
- ½ cup guava nectar, sugar-free
- 5 ice cubes

Directions

1. Take all the ingredients including strawberries, yogurt, banana, guava nectar and ice cubes in a blender and blend until smooth for about 2 minutes.
2. Serve this quick yet delicious smoothie chilled, immediately.

Nutritional Information (for one serving)

Calories: 137

Fat Total: 0.6g

Fat Saturated: 0g

Carbohydrates: 30.1g

Dietary Fiber: 5.4g

Sugars: 19.1g

Protein: 5.5g

Lunch

Baked Meatloaf

Preparation time: 25 minutes   Cooking time: 60 minutes   Serves: 10-12

Ingredients

- 1 (15 ounce) can roasted tomatoes
- 1 cup roasted red peppers
- 1 teaspoon dried oregano
- 4 cloves garlic, minced
- 1 teaspoon cumin

- 3 pound grass-fed ground beef
- 2 organic eggs
- 1 cup coconut flour
- 1 cup tomato paste
- 1 medium onion, finely chopped

Directions

1. Preheat the oven to 350 degrees F.
2. In a food processor, add roasted tomatoes, red peppers, oregano, garlic and cumin. Pulse until well combined mixture is formed.
3. In a bowl, combine together ground beef and eggs.
4. Add coconut flour, tomato paste and onion and mix using your hands.
5. Mix in tomatoes and red peppers mixture until well combined.
6. Place the mixture in a greased loaf pan.
7. Bake in the oven for 45-50 minutes.
8. Broil for 10-12 minutes and serve.

Nutritional Information (for one serving)

Calories: 352

Fat Total: 18.4g

Fat Saturated: 5.1g

Carbohydrates: 18.9g

Dietary Fiber: 4.7g

Sugars: 4.5g

Protein: 26.6g

Dinner

Prawns Salad

Preparation time: 15 minutes   Cooking time: 10 minutes   Serves: 4-6

Ingredients

- 1 tablespoon coconut oil
- 3 bacon slices
- 10 prawns, cooked
- 1 clove garlic, minced
- 2 cups lettuce, chopped
- 6 cherry tomatoes, halved
- 2 tablespoons diced scallions

- Half avocado, sliced
- 1 Quarter red capsicum, sliced
- 1 tablespoon lemon juice
- 1 teaspoon Dijon mustard
- 1 tablespoon olive oil
- Pinch of salt
- Pinch of black pepper

Directions

1. Heat the coconut oil in a saucepan.
2. Add bacon and cook until crispy.
3. Remove the bacon and add prawns and garlic into the pan.
4. Sauté for 2 minutes and remove.
5. In a bowl, add lettuce, tomatoes, scallions, avocado and capsicum and mix.
6. Add in lemon juice, Dijon mustard and olive oil and toss well to combine.
7. Top with prawns, sprinkle with salt and pepper and serve.

Nutritional Information (for one serving)

Calories: 176

Fat Total: 9.6g

Fat Saturated: 3.9g

Carbohydrates: 6.3g

Dietary Fiber: 1.7g

Sugars: 3.5g

Protein: 12.4g

Snack

Fresh Fruit Bowl

Preparation time: 10 minutes   Cooking time: 0 minutes   Serves: 3-4

Ingredients

- 2 apples, peeled, cored and diced
- 1 large banana, peeled and sliced
- ½ cup fresh blueberries
- ½ cup strawberries, halved
- ¼ cup raspberries

Directions

1. Place apples, bananas and blueberries in a bowl.
2. Add in strawberries and raspberries.
3. Toss well and serve.

Nutritional Information (for one serving)

Calories: 98

Fat Total: 0.3g

Fat Saturated: 0g

Carbohydrates: 25.2g

Dietary Fiber: 4.5g

Sugars: 16.5g

Protein: 1g

Dessert

Protein waffles

Preparation time: 40 minutes   Cooking time: 16 minutes   Serving: 4

Ingredients

- ½ cup almond flour

- ½ cup tapioca flour
- ½ cup mocha whey protein powder
- ½ cup vanilla flavoured protein powder
- 1 tablespoons cocoa powder
- 1 teaspoon baking powder
- ¼ teaspoon salt
- 4 eggs
- ¾ cup applesauce, unsweetened
- 1 teaspoon vanilla extract
- 2 tablespoons coconut oil

Directions

1. In a large bowl, combine almond flour, tapioca flour, protein powders, cocoa powder, baking powder and salt.
2. In another bowl, add eggs and beat until light.
3. Add in applesauce, vanilla extract and coconut oil and beat again.
4. Gradually add into the flour mixture and mix until well combined and evenly smooth.
5. Pour ¾ of the batter into a greased waffle iron

and cook for 4 minutes.

6. Follow the same instructions for all the mixture.
7. Remove from the iron and serve.

Nutritional Information (for one serving)

Calories: 198

Fat Total: 13.4g

Fat Saturated: 7.6g

Carbohydrates: 8.5g

Dietary Fiber: 1.4g

Sugars: 5.5g

Protein: 12.6g

Day 7

Breakfast

Chicken Casserole

Preparation Time: 10 minutes   Cooking Time: 1 hour   Serves: 4

Ingredients

- 1 tablespoon coconut oil
- 1 pound boneless chicken, pieces
- 4 eggs, beaten
- 3 turnips, peeled and grated
- 4 scallions, chopped
- Salt and black pepper, to taste

Directions

1. Preheat the oven to 400 degrees F.
2. Lightly grease a casserole dish.
3. In a pan, heat oil on medium heat.
4. Add chicken and sauté for 4 to 5 minutes or till browned.
5. In a large bowl, add all ingredients and mix

well.

6. Place the chicken mixture in prepared casserole dish.
7. Cover and bake for 50 minutes.
8. Uncover and bake for 10 minutes more.
9. Remove from the oven and serve.

Nutritional Information (for one serving)

Calories: 339

Fat Total: 16.2g

Fat Saturated: 6.6g

Carbohydrates: 7.5g

Dietary Fiber: 1.9g

Sugars: 4.4g

Protein: 39.4g

Lunch

Salmon with Spinach & Apple Salad

Prep Time: 15 minutes   Cooking Time: 30 minutes
Serves: 2

Ingredients:

- ½ pound salmon fillets

For salad

- ½ cup baby spinach
- ½ cup lettuce
- ½ cup cabbage, shredded
- 1 tart apple, sliced

For dressing

- 2 tablespoons olive oil
- 2 tablespoons apple cider vinegar
- 1 large shallot, minced
- Salt and black pepper, to taste

Directions:

1. Preheat the oven to 350 degrees F.
2. Place salmon fillet on a baking dish. Season with salt and pepper.
3. Add some water to cover fish. Cover with a foil paper.
4. Bake for 10 minutes. Remove from oven and set aside.

5. In a large bowl, add salad ingredients and mix.
6. In another bowl, add all dressing ingredients and whisk till well combined.
7. Pour dressing over salad and toss to coat.
8. Serve salad with baked fish fillets.

Nutritional Information (for one serving)

Calories: 329

Fat Total: 21.2g

Fat Saturated: 3.0g

Carbohydrates: 14.4g

Dietary Fiber: 2.9g

Sugars: 10.3g

Protein: 22.7g

Dinner

Roasted Beef with Vegetables

Prep Time: 15 minutes   Cooking Time: 35 minutes
Serves: 2

Ingredients:

- 2 tablespoons olive oil
- ½ pound lean beef steak (chuck steak), sliced
- 1 onion, sliced
- 1 tablespoon garlic, minced
- ½ cup asparagus, sliced
- 1 cup zucchini, cubed
- Salt and pepper to taste

Directions:

1. Preheat the oven to 325 degrees F.
2. Heat oil in a pan.
3. Stir in beef and cook for 5 minutes until beef is a little browned.
4. Transfer beef to a baking dish. Add onion, garlic, asparagus and zucchini. Sprinkle with salt and pepper.
5. Place in preheated oven and bake for 30 minutes.

Nutritional Information (for one serving)

Calories: 313

Fat Total: 19.2g

Fat Saturated: 4.1g

Carbohydrates: 9.7g

Dietary Fiber: 2.6g

Sugars: 4g

Protein: 2.1g

Snack

Fruit Salad

Prep Time: 10 minutes   Cooking Time: 0 minutes
Serves: 2

Ingredients:

- 1 apple, peeled and sliced
- ½ cup strawberries, chopped
- ½ cup orange, peeled and sliced
- ½ teaspoon cinnamon

Directions:

1. Combine all the fruits in a bowl, sprinkle with cinnamon and serve.

Nutritional Information (for one serving)

Calories: 81

Fat Total: 0.3g

Fat Saturated: 0g

Carbohydrates: 21.1g

Dietary Fiber: 4.3g

Sugars: 15.5g

Protein: 1g

Dessert

Cherry and Almond Butter Milkshake

Prep Time: 5 minutes   Cooking Time: 0 minutes
Serves: 3

Ingredients:

- 1cup almond milk
- 1 whole banana, frozen
- 8 cherries, frozen
- 2 tablespoons almond butter
- 1 tablespoon honey
- 6-8 Ice cubes

Directions:

1. Place all the ingredients into food processor and blend until smooth and creamy.
2. Serve and enjoy!

Nutritional Information (for one serving)

Calories: 401

Fat Total: 18.9g

Fat Saturated: 13.2g

Carbohydrates: 57.2g

Dietary Fiber: 3.4g

Sugars: 9.8g

Protein: 3.9g

Day 8

Breakfast

Baked Omelette

Prep Time: 10 minutes   Cooking Time: 20 minutes
Serves: 2

Ingredients:

- 3 eggs
- ½ cup coconut milk
- 1 tablespoon fresh chives, minced
- 1 small onion, chopped
- 1 small green bell pepper, deseeded, julienne
- ¼ cup mushrooms, sliced

Directions:

1. Preheat the oven to 400 degrees F. Lightly grease a pie dish.
2. Crack eggs in a bowl, add coconut milk. Season with salt and pepper.
3. Pour eggs in the pie dish. Top with chives, onion, green bell pepper and mushrooms.

4 Bake for 15 to 20 minutes until golden brown.

Nutritional Information (for one serving)

Calories: 261

Fat Total: 21g

Fat Saturated: 14.7g

Carbohydrates: 9.7g

Dietary Fiber: 3g

Sugars: 5.7g

Protein: 10.6g

Dinner

Mushrooms Soup

Prep Time: 10 minutes   Cooking Time: 20 minutes
Serves: 3

Ingredients:

- 2 tablespoons coconut oil
- 1 onion, chopped
- 1 garlic clove, minced
- 2 avocados, sliced

- 1 cup mushrooms, sliced
- 1 red sweet pepper, chopped
- 2 tomatoes, sliced
- sprigs basil leaves
- 3 cups water
- Salt and freshly ground black pepper to taste

Directions:

1. Heat oil in a pan.
2. Add onion and garlic and cook for 3 to 4 minutes until tender.
3. Add avocado, mushrooms, red sweet pepper, tomatoes and basil leaves and continue to cook until the vegetables are tender.
4. Add water and bring to a boil. Cover and cook for 15 minutes.
5. Sprinkle with salt and pepper.
6. When cooked, cool a little, place soup into food processor and blend until smooth and creamy.
7. Reheat, ladle in a soup bowl and serve.

Nutritional Information (for one serving)

Calories: 401

Fat Total: 35.6g

Fat Saturated: 13.4g

Carbohydrates: 21.6g

Dietary Fiber: 11.9g

Sugars: 6.5g

Protein: 4.7g

Snack

Kale Chips

Prep Time: 5 minutes   Cooking Time: 15 minutes
Serves: 2

Ingredients:

- 2 cups kale, remove stems and chop leaves
- 2 tablespoons coconut oil
- ¼ teaspoon salt

Directions:

1. Preheat oven to 350 degrees F.
2. Toss kale in a bowl with oil and sprinkle with

salt.

3. Place kale leaves on a baking sheet, cover sheet with a parchment paper and bake for 10 to 15 minutes or until kale is crispy.

Nutritional Information (for one serving)

Calories: 150

Fat Total: 13.6g

Fat Saturated: 11.8g

Carbohydrates: 7g

Dietary Fiber: 1g

Sugars: 0g

Protein: 2g

Dessert

Pumpkin Muffins

Prep Time: 2 minutes   Cooking Time: 25 minutes
Serves: 5

Ingredients:

- 1½ cups almond flour

- 3 tablespoons coconut flour
- 1 teaspoon baking soda
- 1 teaspoon baking powder
- 1½ teaspoon pumpkin pie spice
- ½ teaspoon ground cinnamon
- 1/8 teaspoon sea salt
- 2 large eggs
- ¾ cup pumpkin puree
- ¼ cup raw honey
- 2 teaspoons almond butter
- 1 tablespoon almonds, toasted and chopped

Directions:

1. Preheat the oven to 400 degrees F.
2. Whisk almond flour, coconut flour, baking soda, baking powder and pumpkin pie spice in a mixing bowl and sprinkle with cinnamon and salt.
3. In another bowl whisk the eggs. Add pumpkin puree, honey and butter.
4. Mix wet ingredients with dry ingredients. Fill the batter in muffin cups until each is almost

full.

5. Sprinkle with almonds.
6. Bake for 20 to 25 minutes or until a toothpick inserted in the centre comes out clean.

Nutritional Information (for one serving)

Calories: 183

Fat Total: 8.6g

Fat Saturated: 1.3g

Carbohydrates: 22.9g

Dietary Fiber: 4g

Sugars: 16g

Protein: 6.1g

Day 9

Breakfast

Omelette Chicken

Prep Time: 5 minutes   Cooking Time: 10 minutes   Serves: 2

Ingredients

- 2 tablespoons coconut oil
- 4 eggs
- ¼ cup red bell pepper, sliced
- 1 tablespoon green chili, chopped
- Salt and pepper to taste
- ½ cup boiled chicken, shredded
- 2 tablespoons parsley, chopped

Directions

1. Beat the eggs in a bowl.
2. Add bell pepper, green chili, chicken, parsley and season to your taste and mix until well combined. In a pan, heat oil on medium heat.
3. Add half of the egg mixture to heated pan.

4. When fully set, fold half of the egg over the filling and cook a minute more.
5. Repeat with the remaining mixture.

Nutritional Information (for one serving)

Calories: 303

Fat Total: 23.5g

Fat Saturated: 14.8g

Carbohydrates: 2.1g

Dietary Fiber: 0g

Sugars: 1.4g

Protein: 21.4g

Lunch

Roasted Fish with Bacon

Prep Time: 10 minutes   Cooking Time: 25minutes
Serves: 4

Ingredients:

- 1 cup almond flour
- 1 cup coconut flour

- Salt and black pepper for seasoning
- 1 pound salmon fillets
- eggs, beaten
- 4 tablespoons almond butter, melted
- 4 slices Bacon
- 1 tablespoons coconut oil

Directions:

1. Preheat the oven to 400 degrees F. Lightly grease a baking dish.
2. Mix almond flour, coconut flour, salt and black pepper in a bowl.
3. In another bowl whisk the eggs.
4. Dip fish fillets in the eggs then into the flour mixture. Set aside.
5. Put bacon slices in a bowl, add oil and season with salt and pepper.
6. Put fish fillets in the baking dish with bacon slices, brush with melted butter and bake for 20-25 minutes.

Nutritional Information (for one serving)

Calories: 294

Fat Total: 35g

Fat Saturated: 9g

Carbohydrates: 20.7g

Dietary Fiber: 11.3g

Sugars: 2.3g

Protein: 39.3g

Dinner

Grilled Chicken with Olives and Tomatoes

Prep Time: 5 minutes   Cooking Time: 10 minutes   Serves: 2

Ingredients:

For topping:
- 2 tablespoons parsley, chopped
- 2 tablespoons basil sprigs
- 1 garlic clove
- 2 sundried tomatoes

- 2 tablespoons olives, pitted
- ¼ cup lemon juice

For Chicken

- 1 skinless and boneless chicken breast
- 2 tablespoons coconut oil
- ¼ teaspoon salt

Directions:

1. Place all the topping ingredients in a food processor and blend until smooth. Set aside.
2. Preheat a grill pan to high.
3. Toss chicken in a bowl with oil and sprinkle with salt.
4. Place chicken on grill pan over medium.
5. Grill for 5 minutes on each side or until well cooked.
6. Serve on a platter drizzled with topping.

Nutritional Information (for one serving)

Calories: 164

Fat Total: 8.4g

Fat Saturated: 6.2g

Carbohydrates: 16.1g

Dietary Fiber: 3.6g

Sugars: 10.5g

Protein: 10.6g

Snack

Green Smoothie

Prep Time: 10 minutes   Cooking Time: 0 minutes
Serves: 2

Ingredients:

- 1 pear, sliced
- 1 apple, sliced
- ½ teaspoon, ginger, chopped
- 2 tablespoons flax seeds
- 2 cups kale leaves
- ¼ cup spinach
- 2 tablespoons lemon juice
- 1 cup water

- Salt and freshly ground black pepper to taste

Directions:

1. Place all the ingredients in food processor and blend until smooth.
2. Season with salt and pepper.
3. Serve and enjoy.

Nutritional Information (for one serving)

Calories: 165

Fat Total: 2.6g

Fat Saturated: 0g

Carbohydrates: 33.5g

Dietary Fiber: 7.4g

Sugars: 17.5g

Protein: 4g

Dessert

Berries with Almonds

Prep Time: 5 minutes   Cooking Time: 0minutes
Serves: 2

Ingredients:

- 1 cup fresh berries
- 2 tablespoons balsamic vinegar
- 2 tablespoons maple syrup
- 1/3 cup almonds, toasted and chopped

Directions:

1. Combine all ingredients in a bowl and serve.

Nutritional Information (for one serving)

Calories: 187

Fat Total: 8.2g

Fat Saturated: 0.6g

Carbohydrates: 25.5g

Dietary Fiber: 4.5g

Sugars: 17.6g

Protein: 3.9g

Day 10

Breakfast

Raspberry Almond Muffins

Prep Time: 10 minutes   Cooking Time: 20 minutes
Serves: 10

Ingredients

- 1cup almond flour, sifted
- ½ teaspoon baking powder
- ½ teaspoon baking soda
- ½ teaspoon salt
- 3 eggs
- 1/3 cup raw honey
- 1/3 cup coconut oil, melted
- ¼ cup almond butter, melted
- ½ teaspoon almond extract
- 1/3 cup almonds, chopped
- 1 cup raspberry, chopped

Directions

1. Preheat the oven to 375 degrees F.
2. In a bowl, mix together almond flour, baking powder, baking soda and salt.
3. In another bowl, mix together eggs, honey, coconut oil, almond butter and almond extract.
4. Mix dry ingredients into wet ingredients.
5. Gently, fold in chopped almonds and raspberry.
6. Dollop the batter in muffin cups 2/3 full.
7. Bake in the oven for 15 to 20 minutes.

Nutritional Information (for one serving)

Calories: 197

Fat Total: 15.2g

Fat Saturated: 7.2g

Carbohydrates: 13.4g

Dietary Fiber: 1.8g

Sugars: 10.2g

Protein: 4.4g

Lunch

Carrot Soup

Prep Time: 15 minutes   Cooking Time: 30 minutes
Serves: 3

Ingredients:

- 2 tablespoons coconut oil
- 2 bay leaves
- 1 onion, sliced
- garlic cloves, minced
- 1 cup carrots, chopped
- 2 turnips, chopped
- 2 sweet potatoes, cubed
- ¼ teaspoon dried thyme
- 2 cups chicken broth
- 2 tablespoons fresh chives, chopped
- Sea salt and freshly ground pepper to taste

Directions:

1. Heat oil in a large soup pan.
2. Stir in bay leaves, onion and garlic and sauté for

few minutes until feel an aroma.

3. Add carrots, turnips, sweet potatoes and dried thyme and continue to cook until the vegetables are tender.
4. Add broth and bring to boil. Cover and cook for 15 to 20 minutes.
5. Discard bay leaves. Pour soup in a food processor and pulse until smooth.
6. Season with salt and pepper.
7. Return to soup pan and let it simmer for 5 minutes.
8. Put soup in a bowl, sprinkle with chives and serve hot.

Nutritional Information (for one serving)

Calories: 278

Fat Total: 10.2g

Fat Saturated: 8.2g

Carbohydrates: 41.3g

Dietary Fiber: 7.2g

Sugars: 7.7g

Protein: 6.1g

Dinner

Fish Curry

Prep Time: 10 minutes   Cooking Time: 20 minutes
Serves: 3

Ingredients:

- 2 tablespoons olive oil
- 1 onion, sliced
- 2 tilapia fillets, strips
- ½ cup coconut milk
- ½ tablespoon red curry paste
- 1 teaspoon lemon juice
- 1 banana, sliced
- 1 tablespoon almonds, chopped
- ½ cup fresh cilantro, chopped
- 1 lemon, sliced
- Pinch of salt and freshly ground black pepper

Directions:

1. Heat oil in a large frying pan.
2. Stir in onion and tilapia fillets, cook for 8 to 10 minutes until tilapia is cooked.
3. Add coconut milk, red curry paste and lemon juice and cook for 2 minutes.
4. Add banana slices and almonds and cook for 5 minutes. season with salt and pepper
5. Sprinkle with cilantro and lemon slices and serve.

Nutritional Information (for one serving)

Calories: 307

Fat Total: 21.3g

Fat Saturated: 10.5g

Carbohydrates: 15.7g

Dietary Fiber: 3.2g

Sugars: 7.7g

Protein: 16.1g

Snack

Strawberry & banana Smoothie

Prep Time: 10 minutes   Cooking Time: 0 minutes
Serves: 2

Ingredients

- 1 cup watermelon, chunks
- 1 banana, sliced
- 2 strawberries
- ½ cup coconut milk

Directions:

1. Place all the ingredients in food processor and blend until smooth and creamy.
2. Serve and enjoy.

Nutritional Information (for one serving)

Calories: 217

Fat Total: 14.4g

Fat Saturated: 12.8g

Carbohydrates: 23.4g

Dietary Fiber: 3.6g

Sugars: 14.3g

Protein: 2.5g

Dessert

Apple Pudding

Prep Time: 3 minutes   Cooking Time: 5 minutes
Serves: 3

Ingredients

- 3 tablespoons coconut oil
- 1 cup coconut milk
- 2 tablespoons raw honey
- 2 apples, sliced
- 1 teaspoon cinnamon

Directions

1. Heat oil in a large pan.
2. Add coconut milk, honey and apples cook for 5 minutes until apples are tender. Remove from the heat. Let it cool.
3. Place apple mixture in a food processor and

pulse until smooth.

4. Sprinkle with cinnamon and serve with fresh fruits.

Nutritional Information (for one serving)

Calories: 409

Fat Total: 32.9g

Fat Saturated: 28.7g

Carbohydrates: 33.4g

Dietary Fiber: 5.1g

Sugars: 26.8g

Protein: 2.2g

Day 11

Breakfast

Delicious Pancakes

Prep Time: 5 minutes   Cooking Time: 10 minutes   Serves: 2

Ingredients

- 1 cup almond flour
- 1 tablespoon coconut flour
- ¼ teaspoon salt
- ½ cup homemade applesauce
- ¼ cup almond milk
- 2 eggs
- ½ teaspoon nutmeg, grated
- ½ cup fresh berries

Directions

1. In a large bowl, add all ingredients and mix till well combined.
2. Heat the non-stick greased frying pan.
3. Dollop ½ cupful of the batter into the heated pan.

4. Cook for 4 to 5 minutes from each side.
5. Repeat the same instruction for the remaining batter and serve.

Nutritional Information (for one serving)

Calories: 250

Fat Total: 19.2g

Fat Saturated: 8.5g

Carbohydrates: 11.5g

Dietary Fiber: 4.8g

Sugars: 4.8g

Protein: 10g

Lunch

Prawns with Tomato Sauce

Prep Time: 5 minutes   Cooking Time: 10 minutes
Serves: 2

Ingredients:

- 2 tablespoons olive oil
- 1 red onion, chopped

- 1 cloves garlic, minced
- ½ pound prawns
- 2 medium tomatoes, chopped
- ½ teaspoon cayenne pepper
- 1 teaspoon oregano
- 2 tablespoons celery, chopped
- 2 tablespoons capers
- ½ teaspoon sea salt
- ½ teaspoon black pepper

Directions:

1. Heat oil in a large frying pan.
2. Stir in onion and garlic and cook for few minutes until you feel an aroma.
3. Add prawns and tomatoes and cook for 6-7 minutes until prawns are tender.
4. Sprinkle with cayenne pepper, oregano, celery and capers, season with salt and pepper and serve.

Nutritional Information (for one serving)

Calories: 309

Fat Total: 16.4g

Fat Saturated: 2.7g

Carbohydrates: 13.7g

Dietary Fiber: 3.6g

Sugars: 5.7g

Protein: 28.0g

Dinner

Sautéed Juicy Pork Tenderloin with Apple

Prep Time: 10 minutes   Cooking Time: 35-40 minutes   Serves: 2

Ingredients:

- 1 tablespoon coconut oil
- 1 onion, chopped
- ½ pound pork tenderloin, sliced
- 1 apple, sliced
- 2 tablespoons rosemary

- 1 cup beef broth
- 2 tablespoons apple cider vinegar
- Salt and pepper to taste

Directions:

1. Heat oil in a large saucepan over medium.
2. Stir in onion and sauté until onion is translucent. Add pork and cook for few minutes until pork is a little browned.
3. Add apple, rosemary and beef broth, cover and continue to cook for 30 minutes until the pork is tender and gravy thickens a little.
4. Drizzle vinegar, season with salt and pepper and serve.

Nutritional Information (for one serving)

Calories: 324

Fat Total: 12.0g

Fat Saturated: 7.7g

Carbohydrates: 20.3g

Dietary Fiber: 4.7g

Sugars: 12.1g

Protein: 32.8g

Snack

Banana Chips

Prep Time: 5 minutes   Cooking Time: 30 minutes
Serves: 2

Ingredients:

- 2 bananas, cut into 1/8 inch slices
- 2 tablespoons lemon juice
- 2 tablespoons nutmeg

Directions

1. Preheat oven to 300 degrees F. Line a baking sheet with parchment paper.
2. In a medium bowl, add all ingredients and mix well.
3. Spread banana slices evenly over baking sheet in a single layer. Make sure banana slices are at least ½ inch apart.
4. Bake for 30 minutes or until banana slices are nicely golden in colour.

5. Remove from oven, let cool a little and then serve.

Nutritional Information (for one serving)

Calories: 145

Fat Total: 3.1g

Fat Saturated: 2.0g

Carbohydrates: 30.8g

Dietary Fiber: 4.6g

Sugars: 16.7g

Protein: 1.8g

Dessert

Coconut Bread

Prep Time: 5 minutes   Cooking Time: 30 minutes
Serves: 4

Ingredients:

- 1 cup coconut flour, sifted
- ½ teaspoon baking soda
- ½ teaspoon salt
- eggs, lightly whisked

- 1 tablespoon maple syrup
- ½ cup butter, melted

Directions:

1. Preheat the oven to 350 degrees F. Lightly, grease and flour a loaf pan.
2. In a bowl, mix flour, baking soda and salt. In another bowl, whisk eggs with maple syrup and butter.
3. Add flour mixture to egg mixture and mix till well combined.
4. Place the batter in the loaf pan. Bake for 25 to 30 minutes or until a toothpick inserted in the center comes out clean.
5. Remove from oven. Let it cool. Cut into slices and serve with coconut butter.

Nutritional Information (for one serving)

Calories: 435

Fat Total: 32.6g

Fat Saturated: 17.6g

Carbohydrates: 19.9g

Dietary Fiber: 10.0g

Sugars: 5.5g

Protein: 12.5g

Day 12

Breakfast

Jalapeno Scrambled Eggs with Cherry Tomatoes

Prep Time: 5 minutes   Cooking Time: 15 minutes   Serves: 3

Ingredients:

- large eggs
- 2 egg whites
- Salt and black pepper, to taste
- 1 teaspoon dried thyme
- 3 tablespoons almond butter
- 1 cup cherry tomatoes, halved
- 2 small jalapenos, seeded and chopped
- 4 scallions, chopped

Directions

1. In a bowl, add eggs, egg whites, salt, black pepper and thyme and whisk well.

2. Melt butter in a frying pan over medium high heat.

3. Add tomatoes and jalapenos and cook for 2 to 3 minutes.

4. Add egg mixture and cook for 4 to 5 minutes until eggs are done completely, stirring occasionally.

5. Stir in scallions and cook for 1 to 2 minutes.

Nutritional Information (for one serving)

Calories: 227

Fat Total: 15.9g

Fat Saturated: 3.0g

Carbohydrates: 7.7g

Dietary Fiber: 2.1g

Sugars: 2.8g

Protein: 15.2g

Lunch

Sautéed Leeks with Salmon

Prep Time: 10 minutes   Cooking Time: 30 minutes
Serves: 2

Ingredients:

- 2 tablespoons almond butter
- ½ cup chopped leeks
- 2 tablespoons chopped celery
- 2 carrots, sliced
- 2 salmon fillets, cut into strips
- 2 tablespoons lemon juice
- Salt and pepper to taste

Directions:

1. Melt 1 tablespoon butter in a sauté pan over medium.
2. Stir in carrots and cook for 5 minutes, stirring often. Add leeks and celery and continue cooking for 5 minutes more or until carrots are crisply tender. Remove vegetables into a plate and set aside.

3. Heat remaining butter in the same pan and add salmon. Let simmer, stirring occasionally, for 15 minutes until fish is cooked through. Add in sautéed vegetables and stir for 2 minutes until vegetables are heated through.
4. Drizzle lemon juice, season with salt and pepper and serve.

Nutritional Information (for one serving)

Calories: 380

Fat Total: 20.4g

Fat Saturated: 2.6g

Carbohydrates: 12.3g

Dietary Fiber: 2.9g

Sugars: 4.2g

Protein: 39.0g

Dinner

Spicy Mixed Vegetable Curry

Prep Time: 10 minutes   Cooking Time: 30 minutes
Serves: 2

Ingredients:

- 1 tablespoon coconut oil
- 1 onion, chopped
- 3 clove garlic, minced
- 1 teaspoon fresh ginger, grated
- ¼ cup carrots, cubed
- ¼ cup broccoli, cubed
- ¼ cup zucchini, cube
- ¼ cup mushrooms
- ½ cup coconut milk
- 1 teaspoon ground cumin
- ½ teaspoon ground coriander
- ½ teaspoon ground turmeric
- ¼ teaspoon cayenne pepper
- ¼ teaspoon ground nutmeg
- Salt and pepper for seasoning

Directions:

1. Heat oil in a large frying pan.
2. Stir in onion, garlic and ginger and cook for a

few minutes until onion is translucent.

3. Add carrots, broccoli, zucchini and mushrooms and continue to cook for 10 minutes until vegetables are crisply tender.
4. Add coconut milk, sprinkle cumin, coriander, turmeric, cayenne pepper and nutmeg. Season with salt and pepper and cook for 5 to 8 minutes until the gravy thickens.
5. Serve hot sprinkled with freshly chopped coriander.

Nutritional Information (for one serving)

Calories: 250

Fat Total: 21.7g

Fat Saturated: 18.7g

Carbohydrates: 14.3g

Dietary Fiber: 3.9g

Sugars: 5.6g

Protein: 3.5g

Snack

Baked Apple

Prep Time: 5 minutes   Cooking Time: 30 minutes
Serves: 1

Ingredients:
- 2 apples, round slices
- 1 cinnamon stick
- 2 cups fresh apple juice
- Pinch of salt and pepper

Directions:
1. Preheat the oven to 350 degrees F.
2. Lightly grease a baking dish.
3. Combine all ingredients in a mixing bowl and season with salt and pepper.
4. Cover and marinate overnight.
5. Spread apple on a baking dish.
6. Bake for 25 to 30 minutes or until browned.

Nutritional Information (for one serving)
Calories: 214

Fat Total: 0.3g

Fat Saturated: 0.0g

Carbohydrates: 54.9g

Dietary Fiber: 5.2g

Sugars: 46.0g

Protein: 0.2g

Dessert

Coconut Whipped Cream

Prep Time: 5 minutes   Refrigerating Time: 2-3 hours   Serves: 2

Ingredients:

- 1 cup coconut cream
- 1 cup coconut milk
- 1/8 teaspoon cinnamon
- 1/8 teaspoon vanilla extract
- 1 teaspoon ground nutmeg

Directions:

1. Place all the ingredients in food processor and blend until smooth and creamy.

2. Pour coconut cream in 2 cups and refrigerate for at least 2 to3 hours.
3. Serve and enjoy!

Nutritional Information (for one serving)

Calories: 559

Fat Total: 57.6g

Fat Saturated: 51.0g

Carbohydrates: 14.0g

Dietary Fiber: 5.6g

Sugars: 8.4g

Protein: 5.6g

Day 13

Breakfast

Eggs with Spicy Tomato Sauce

Prep Time: 10 minutes   Cooking Time: 15 minutes
Serves: 2

Ingredients:

- 2 tablespoons coconut oil
- 1 medium onion, chopped
- cloves garlic, minced
- 1 red bell pepper, deseeded, julienne
- 1 jalapeno pepper, deseeded, julienne
- ½ cup tomatoes, chopped
- 1 teaspoon cumin
- 2 large eggs
- Seasons with salt and pepper
- 2 tablespoons parsley, chopped

Directions:

1. Heat oil in a large frying pan.

2. Stir in onion and garlic and cook for few minutes until little browned.
3. Add red bell pepper, jalapeno and tomatoes and continue to cook until the vegetables are tender.
4. Sprinkle with cumin and salt.
5. Crack eggs in a bowl and season with salt and pepper.
5. Pour eggs in the frying pan.
6. Cook for 5 minutes or until slightly golden. Flip and cook other side until eggs are done.
7. Sprinkle with parsley and serve.

Nutritional Information (for one serving)

Calories: 254

Fat Total: 19.2g

Fat Saturated: 13.4g

Carbohydrates: 14.0g

Dietary Fiber: 3.4g

Sugars: 6.4g

Protein: 8.6g

Lunch

Thai Fish Curry

Prep Time: 10 minutes   Cooking Time: 25 minutes
Serves: 2

Ingredients:

- ½ cup coconut milk
- 1 cup fresh basil leaves
- 4 tablespoons Thai curry paste
- 2 tablespoons olive oil
- 2 tilapia fillets
- 1 large red bell peppers, deseeded, julienne
- 1 onion, sliced
- ¼ cup scallions, sliced
- 2 tablespoons fish sauce
- Salt and freshly ground black pepper to taste

Directions:

1. Place coconut milk, basil leaves and Thai curry paste into food processor and blend until smooth.

2. Heat oil in a large pan. Stir in tilapia fillets and cook for 5 minutes on each side until little browned. Remove tilapia in a plate and set aside.
3. Add red bell peppers, onion and scallions in the same pan and cook until the vegetables are tender.
4. Add coconut milk mixture and cook for 5 minutes until thickens.
5. Add in reserved fish fillets and simmer until tilapia is heated through.
6. Drizzle fish sauce, season with salt and pepper and serve.

Nutritional Information (for one serving)

Calories: 441

Fat Total: 29.7g

Fat Saturated: 15.1g

Carbohydrates: 21.1g

Dietary Fiber: 4.7g

Sugars: 10.6g

Protein: 25.3g

Dinner

Grilled Chicken with Olive and Tomato Topping

Prep Time: 5 minutes   Cooking Time: 10 minutes   Serves: 2

Ingredients:

For topping:

- 2 tablespoons parsley, chopped
- 2 tablespoons basil sprigs
- 1 garlic clove
- 2 sundried tomatoes
- 2 tablespoons olives, pitted
- ¼ cup lemon juice

For Chicken

- 1 skinless and boneless chicken breast
- 2 tablespoons coconut oil
- ¼ teaspoon salt

Directions:

1. Place all the topping ingredients in a food processor and blend until smooth. Set aside.
2. Preheat a grill pan to high.
3. Toss chicken in a bowl with oil and sprinkle with salt.
4. Place chicken on grill pan over medium.
5. Grill for 5 minutes on each side or until well cooked (to your desired doneness). Serve on a platter drizzled with topping.

Nutritional Information (for one serving)

Calories: 338

Fat Total: 17.9g

Fat Saturated: 12.6g

Carbohydrates: 32.1g

Dietary Fiber: 7.2g

Sugars: 21.0g

Protein: 20.2g

Snack

Watermelon & Kiwi with Fresh Herbs

Prep Time: 10 minutes   Cooking Time: 0 minutes
Serves: 2

Ingredients:

- 4 cups watermelon
- 1 kiwi, chopped
- ½ teaspoon fresh oregano, chopped
- ½ teaspoon fresh cilantro, chopped
- ½ teaspoon fresh mint leaves
- ½ teaspoon fresh basil leaves, chopped
- ½ teaspoon fresh parsley, chopped
- 1/8 teaspoon salt
- Pinch of ground black pepper

Directions:

1. Toss all ingredients in a mixing bowl and season with salt and pepper.

Nutritional Information (for one serving)

Calories: 116

Fat Total: 0.7g

Fat Saturated: 0.0g

Carbohydrates: 28.9g

Dietary Fiber: 2.6g

Sugars: 22.3g

Protein: 2.4g

Dessert

Creamy Banana Treat with Cranberries and Coconut milk

Prep Time: 5 minutes   Cooking Time: 0 minutes
Serves: 2

Ingredients:

- 1 large banana, sliced
- 2 tablespoons almond butter
- 2 tablespoons coconut milk
- ½ cup cranberries
- Pinch of cinnamon

Directions:

1. Combine bananas with almond butter and co-

conut milk in a large bowl.

2. Add cranberries on top and sprinkle with cinnamon before serving.

Nutritional Information (for one serving)

Calories: 208

Fat Total: 12.9g

Fat Saturated: 4.1g

Carbohydrates: 22.2g

Dietary Fiber: 3.9g

Sugars: 9.8g

Protein: 4.6g

Day 14

Breakfast

Breakfast Casserole

Prep Time: 10 minutes   Cooking Time: 40 minutes
Serves: 3

Ingredients:

- ¼ pound bacon, diced
- 2 tablespoons coconut oil plus 1 teaspoon coconut oil
- 3 eggs, whisked
- 1 small onion, chopped
- 1 red bell pepper, deseeded, julienne
- 1 tomato, deseeded, sliced
- 1 tablespoon cilantro
- ½ cup coconut cream
- Salt and pepper to taste

Directions:

1. Preheat oven to 350 degrees F and lightly spray a baking dish with cooking spray.

2. Heat 1 teaspoon oil in a skillet and sauté onion for 3 minutes or until softened. Add in bacon and cook stirring for 5 minutes.
3. Remove bacon and onion mixture into a bowl. Add rest of the ingredients in bowl and seasons with salt and pepper.
4. Place mixture over baking dish.
5. Bake for 30 to 35 minutes or till golden browned.

Nutritional Information (for one serving)

Calories: 463

Fat Total: 38.9g

Fat Saturated: 22.9g

Carbohydrates: 8.4g

Dietary Fiber: 2.4g

Sugars: 4.8g

Protein: 21.3g

Lunch

Grilled Spicy Beef

Prep Time: 5 minutes   Cooking Time: 10 minutes
Serves: 2

Ingredients:

- ¼ pound sirloin beef roast, sliced
- 2 tablespoons olive oil
- 2 tablespoons lemon juice
- 1 clove garlic, finely chopped
- ¼ teaspoon cayenne pepper
- 1 teaspoon chili powder
- 1 teaspoon green chili, chopped
- ½ teaspoon oregano
- ¼ teaspoon salt
- ½ teaspoon freshly ground black pepper

Directions:

1. Combine all ingredients in a bowl and mix together.
2. Leave marinated for at least 2 hours.

3. Preheat a grill pan to high.
4. Place beef slices on grill pan over medium.
5. Grill for 5 minutes on each side or until to your desired doneness.

Nutritional Information (for one serving)

Calories: 195

Fat Total: 17.0g

Fat Saturated: 3.2g

Carbohydrates: 2.9g

Dietary Fiber: 0.9g

Sugars: 0.5g

Protein: 9.6g

Dinner

Sweet & Salty Chocolate Bark

Prep Time: 2 minutes Cooking Time: 3 minute
Serves: 4

Ingredients:

- ½ cup dark chocolate, chopped

- ½ cup dried cherries, chopped
- 1 cup pecans
- ¼ teaspoon salt

Directions:

1. Melt chocolate in a saucepan.
2. Stir in cherries, pecans and salt and cook for few seconds.
3. Spread chocolate mixture on a baking dish with a spatula.
4. Refrigerate for at least 1 hour until set.
5. Serve and enjoy!

Nutritional Information (for one serving)

Calories: 221

Fat Total: 16.0g

Fat Saturated: 5.2g

Carbohydrates: 18.1g

Dietary Fiber: 2.1g

Sugars: 11.4g

Protein: 2.9g

Snack

Cocoa Almond Squares

Prep Time: 5 minutes   Cooking Time: 18 minutes
Serves: 4

Ingredients:

- 1 cup almond flour
- 1 tablespoon coconut flour
- 3 tablespoon cocoa powder
- ¼ teaspoon salt
- 1 egg white
- ¼ cup raw honey
- 1 tablespoon coconut oil

Directions

1. Preheat oven to 350 degrees F.
2. In a medium bowl, add almond flour, coconut flour, cocoa powder and salt and mix well.
3. In another bowl, whisk egg white. Add honey and coconut oil and mix again.
4. Mix wet ingredients with dry ingredients until smooth dough is formed.

5. Roll out dough onto a piece of parchment paper. Sandwich it between two sheets and the using a sharp knife slice into squares.
6. Bake for 15 to 18 minutes.

Nutritional Information (for one serving)

Calories: 154

Fat Total: 7.15g

Fat Saturated: 3.5g

Carbohydrates: 22.2g

Dietary Fiber: 2.6g

Sugars: 17.9g

Protein: 3.9.g

Dessert

Chocolate Pudding

Prep Time: 1 hour   Cooking Time: 0 minutes
Serves: 3

Ingredients:

- 2 tablespoons cocoa powder

- 1 avocado, chopped
- ½ cup almond milk
- 4 tablespoons raw honey
- 1 teaspoon vanilla extract

Directions:

1. Place all the ingredients into food processor and blend until smooth and creamy.
2. Refrigerator for 1 hour until set.
3. Serve chilled and enjoy!

Nutritional Information (for one serving)

Calories: 320

Fat Total: 23.1g

Fat Saturated: 10.2g

Carbohydrates: 27.8g

Dietary Fiber: 6.5g

Sugars: 25.0g

Protein: 2.9g

Conclusion

So if you are craving for a healthy and fantastic lifestyle then this cookbook is surely for you. This book, consisting of 14 days plan of this amazing ketogenic diet is a perfect start to adopt this plan. The simplicity of the recipes allows you to have a confidence start. The nutritional analysis with each recipe in the book helps you to keep an eye on the nutritional intake of each meal you have. This book provides you an idea of this meal plan with a good explanation of this diet so that you may try designing your own ketogenic meal plan later. In short, this cookbook is worth a try. Grab this book and open new doors of healthiness and fitness.

BONUS: Free Books & Special Offers

I want to thank you again for downloading this book! I would like to give you access to a great service that will e-mail you notifications when we have FREE books available. You will have FREE access to some great titles before they get marked at the normal retail price that everyone else will pay. This is a no strings attached offer simply for being a great customer.

*Simply go to www.globalizedhealing.com to get started.

Copyright 2014 by Globalized Healing, LLC **- All rights reserved.**

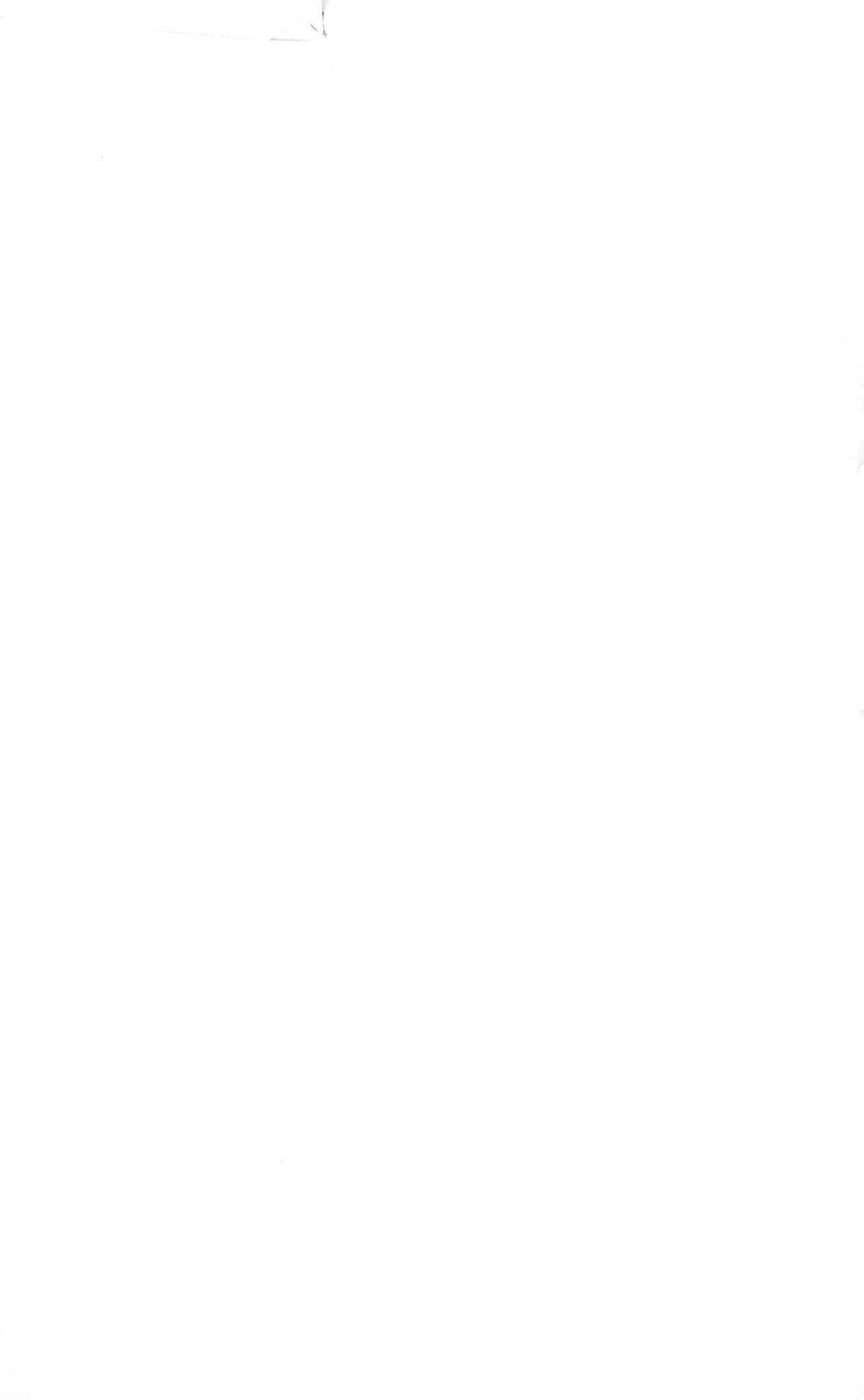

Made in the USA
San Bernardino, CA
11 September 2016